PRENATAL DIETS: NUTRITIONAL GUIDE FOR EXPECTING MOTHERS

Copyright Material

All rights reserved. No part of this publication may be reproduced, distributed, or transmitted in any form or by any means, including photocopying, recording, or methods, without the prior written permission of the publisher, except in the case of brief questions embodied in critical reviews and certain other non-commercial users permitted by copyright law.

About the book

"Prenatal Diets" by Jane Lordson is a comprehensive guide that offers valuable insights and practical advice on nutrition during pregnancy. With a focus on promoting maternal and fetal health, Jane combines her expertise as a nurse with her passion for advocating for healthy pregnancies to create a resource that is both informative and empowering.

The book covers essential nutrients needed during pregnancy, debunks common myths about diet and pregnancy, and provides practical tips for managing pregnancy symptoms through nutrition. Jane's evidence-based approach ensures that readers receive accurate information to make informed decisions about their diet during this crucial time.

One of the standout features of "Prenatal Diets" is the inclusion of practical meal plans and recipes tailored to each stage of pregnancy. These resources make it easy for expecting mothers to incorporate the necessary nutrients into their daily meals, ensuring that both mother and baby receive the nourishment they need for optimal health.

Jane's compassionate tone and dedication to supporting expecting mothers shine through in every chapter of the book. Her commitment to empowering women with the knowledge and tools they need to make healthy choices sets "Prenatal Diets" apart as a trusted resource in the field of prenatal nutrition.

Overall, "Prenatal Diets" is a must-read for anyone looking to prioritize their health and the health of their baby during pregnancy. Jane Lordson's expertise and passion make this book an invaluable resource for expecting mothers seeking guidance on how to nourish themselves and their growing baby throughout pregnancy.

About the author

Jane Lordson is a dedicated nurse and passionate advocate for maternal and fetal health. With years of experience working in the field of obstetrics and gynecology, Jane has witnessed firsthand the profound impact that proper nutrition can have on the health and well-being of both mother and baby.

Drawing on her expertise in nursing and her deep commitment to promoting healthy pregnancies, Jane has authored the insightful and informative book "Prenatal Diets." This comprehensive guide is a testament to Jane's dedication to empowering expecting mothers with the knowledge and tools they need to optimize their diet during pregnancy.

Through her book, Jane shares evidence-based information on the essential nutrients needed during pregnancy, debunks common myths surrounding diet and pregnancy, and offers practical tips for managing pregnancy symptoms through nutrition. Her emphasis on the long-term health implications of maternal nutrition underscores her belief in the importance of establishing healthy eating habits early on.

Jane's expertise shines through in the practical meal plans and recipes she provides, tailored to each stage of pregnancy. Her compassionate approach and unwavering commitment to supporting expecting mothers make "Prenatal Diets" a must-read for anyone seeking guidance on how to nourish themselves and their baby throughout pregnancy.

Jane Lordson's dedication to maternal and fetal health is evident in every page of "Prenatal Diets," making her a trusted authority in the field of prenatal nutrition.

Table of content

Chapter 1: Introduction to prenatal nutrition

- Overview of key nutrients needed during pregnancy   7
- Importance of proper nutrition during pregnancy   9
- Common myths and misconceptions about prenatal diet   10
- Maternal nutrition and fetal development   12
- The role of prenatal nutrition in preventing birth defects   13

Chapter 2: Nutrient needs during pregnancy

- Essential nutrients for a healthy pregnancy   16
- Recommended daily intake of micronutrients during pregnancy   17
- Important hydration and adequate water intake during pregnancy   19
- Role of prenatal vitamins in adequate water intake during pregnancy   21
- Sources of key nutrients in a prenatal diet   23

Chapter 3: Meal planning for pregnancy

- Tips for creating a balanced meal plan during pregnancy   25
- Importance of variety and diversity in food choices during pregnancy   27
- Meal plans for each trimester   29
- Incorporating nutrient dense foods into a prenatal diet   31
- Strategies for managing craving and aversions   32

Chapter 4: Food safety during pregnancy

- Safe food handling and preparation during pregnancy   35
- Common food borne illnesses to be aware of during pregnancy   36
- Potential risks associated with certain foods   38
- List of food to avoid or limit during pregnancy   41
- Alternatives and substitute for restricted foods   42
- Safe food preparation and storage during pregnancy   44

Chapter 5: Managing morning sickness and food aversion

- Coping with morning sickness   46
- Nutrient-dense foods good for the body   47
- Tips for staying hydrated and maintaining adequate food nutrition   49

-   Herbal remedies and natural solutions for managing morning sickness. 50

Chapter 6: Gestational diabetes and prenatal nutrition
-   Gestational diabetes and its effect on pregnancy   53
-   Managing gestational diabetes   55
-   Monitoring blood sugar level   57

Chapter 7: Vegetarian and vegan diets during pregnancy
-   Meeting nutrient needs on a vegan diet   59
-   Plant –based sources of nutrients for pregnancy   60
-   Potential supplements to consider for vegan mothers   62

Chapter 8: Weight management during pregnant
-   Healthy weight gain for pregnancy   64
-   Managing weight gain and promoting healthy pregnancy   66
-   Importance of physical activity and balanced diet   67

Chapter 9: Postpartum nutrition and breastfeeding
-   Nutrition needs during the postpartum period   68
-   Tips for supporting breastfeeding through nutrition   79
-   Transition back to a regular diet after pregnancy   71

Conclusion   73

CHAPTER 1: INTRODUCTION TO PRENATAL NUTRITION

Introduction:

Pregnancy is a transformative and crucial time in a woman's life, marked by the incredible journey of nurturing and growing a new life within. One of the most vital aspects of a healthy pregnancy is proper prenatal nutrition. The food and nutrients consumed during pregnancy play a significant role in supporting the growth and development of the fetus, as well as maintaining the health and well-being of the mother.

Prenatal nutrition is not only about eating for two but also about ensuring that both the mother and baby receive the essential nutrients they need for optimal health. A well-balanced and nutrient-rich diet during pregnancy can help prevent birth defects, support healthy fetal growth, reduce the risk of complications during childbirth, and promote overall well-being for both mother and baby.

In this guide, we will explore the importance of prenatal nutrition, the specific nutrient needs during pregnancy, meal planning tips, foods to avoid, and strategies for managing common challenges such as morning sickness and food aversions. By understanding the role of nutrition in pregnancy and making informed choices about food and lifestyle habits, expectant mothers can lay a strong foundation for a healthy pregnancy and the well-being of their growing baby.

Overview of key nutrients needed during pregnancy.

During pregnancy, the body's nutrient needs increase to support the growth and development of the fetus, as well as to maintain the health of the mother. Here is an overview of key nutrients that are essential during pregnancy:

1. Folic Acid (Folate): Folic acid is a B vitamin that is crucial for preventing neural tube defects in the developing fetus, such as spina bifida. It is recommended that pregnant women consume 600-800 micrograms of folic acid daily, ideally starting before conception and continuing throughout the first trimester.

2. Iron: Iron is important for the production of red blood cells and to prevent anemia in both the mother and baby. Pregnant women need more iron to support the increased blood volume and to provide oxygen to the fetus. Lean meats, chicken, fish, lentils, and fortified cereals are good sources of iron.

3. Calcium: Calcium is essential for building strong bones and teeth in the developing baby. Pregnant women should aim to consume 1,000 milligrams of calcium daily, which can be obtained from dairy products, leafy greens, fortified foods, and supplements if needed.

4. Vitamin D: Vitamin D is important for calcium absorption and bone health. Pregnant women should aim to get 600-800 IU of vitamin D daily through sunlight exposure, fortified foods, and supplements.

5. Omega-3 Fatty Acids: Omega-3 fatty acids, specifically DHA (docosahexaenoic acid), are important for brain and eye development in the fetus. Good sources of omega-3s include fatty fish like salmon, walnuts, flaxseeds, and fortified foods.

6. Protein: Protein is essential for the growth and development of tissues in both the mother and baby. Pregnant women should aim to consume about 71 grams of protein per day from sources like lean meats, poultry, fish, eggs, dairy, legumes, nuts, and seeds.

7. Vitamins A, C, E, and B Vitamins: These vitamins play various roles in supporting overall health, immune function, and fetal development. Eating a variety of fruits, vegetables, whole grains, nuts, seeds, and lean proteins can help ensure an adequate intake of these essential vitamins.

8. Water: Staying hydrated is crucial during pregnancy to support the increased blood volume, amniotic fluid, and overall health. It is recommended that pregnant women try to consume 8 to 10 glasses of water a day.

In addition to these key nutrients, it's important for pregnant women to focus on a well-balanced diet that includes a variety of nutrient-dense foods to meet their increased energy needs during pregnancy. Consulting with a healthcare provider or a registered dietitian can help ensure that individual nutrient needs are met through diet and possibly supplementation when necessary.

Importance of proper nutrition during pregnancy

Proper nutrition throughout pregnancy is critical to the health and well-being of both the mother and the developing baby. Here are some key reasons why maintaining a healthy and balanced diet is essential during pregnancy:

1. Fetal Development: The nutrients consumed by the mother play a vital role in supporting the growth and development of the fetus. Adequate intake of essential nutrients such as folic acid, iron, calcium, protein, and omega-3 fatty acids is important for the formation of organs, tissues, and bones in the developing baby.

2. Reduced Risk of Birth Defects: A well-balanced diet that includes important nutrients like folic acid can help reduce the risk of neural tube defects, such as spina bifida, in the developing baby. Iron deficiency can also lead to anemia in both the mother and baby if not addressed through proper nutrition.

3. Maternal Health: Proper nutrition during pregnancy is essential for maintaining the health and well-being of the mother. Adequate intake of nutrients like iron, calcium, and protein can help prevent maternal complications such as anemia, preeclampsia, and gestational diabetes.

4. Healthy Weight Gain: Pregnancy is a time when weight gain is expected and necessary for the growth of the baby. However, excessive weight gain or inadequate weight gain can lead to complications such as preterm birth, macrosomia (large birth weight), and cesarean delivery. A balanced diet that meets the increased energy needs of pregnancy can help support healthy weight gain.

5. Energy Levels: Pregnancy can be physically demanding, and proper nutrition is essential for maintaining energy levels and supporting overall health. Consuming a variety of nutrient-dense foods can help prevent fatigue, improve mood, and support the body's physiological changes during pregnancy.

6. Immune Function: A well-nourished body is better equipped to support a healthy immune system, which is important during pregnancy to protect both the mother and baby from infections and illnesses.

7. Postpartum Recovery: Proper nutrition during pregnancy can also have long-term benefits for postpartum recovery and breastfeeding. Adequate intake of nutrients like calcium, protein, and iron can support healing after childbirth and provide essential nutrients for breastfeeding.

It's important for pregnant women to focus on eating a variety of nutrient-dense foods from all food groups to ensure they are meeting their increased nutrient needs during pregnancy. Consulting with a healthcare provider or a registered dietitian can help develop a personalized nutrition plan that meets individual needs and supports a healthy pregnancy and optimal fetal development.

Common myths and misconceptions about prenatal diets

There are some prevalent myths and misconceptions about prenatal diets that can cause confusion and possibly harm the health of both the mother and the developing baby. Here are several important ways that maternal diet affects fetal development:

1. Eating for Two: One of the most popular myths regarding prenatal nutrition is that pregnant women must consume much more food since they are "eating for two." In truth, calorie requirements during pregnancy only increase modestly in the second and third trimesters, and it is more necessary to prioritize food quality over quantity. Overeating can cause excessive weight gain, increasing the risk of pregnancy problems.

2. Avoiding Weight Gain: Some women believe that avoiding weight gain during pregnancy is essential for keeping their figure. However, weight increase is an expected and required aspect of a healthy pregnancy. Inadequate weight gain can

lead to poor fetal growth and development, whereas excessive weight gain can raise the risk of problems such as gestational diabetes and high blood pressure.

3. "Eating Clean": The term "eating clean" has become popular in recent years, emphasizing the intake of entire, unprocessed foods. While this is a generally healthy approach, pregnant women may interpret it as avoiding specific food groups or critical nutrients. To satisfy the increased nutrient needs during pregnancy, it is critical to have a well-balanced diet rich in foods from all food categories.

4. Avoiding Fish: There is a common myth that pregnant women should avoid all fish due to mercury exposure. While certain fish have high levels of mercury, others are enriched in omega-3 fatty acids, which are essential for prenatal brain development. Pregnant women can safely eat low-mercury fish like salmon, sardines, and trout in moderation.

5. Vegetarian or Vegan Diets: Another prevalent misconception is that vegetarian or vegan diets are inappropriate for pregnancy. While these diets can be healthful if properly planned, pregnant women who follow vegetarian or vegan diets must be especially careful to receive enough protein, iron, calcium, vitamin B12, Plant-based or supplemented omega-3 fatty acids.

6. Cravings as Nutrient Deficiencies: It is widely held that pregnant cravings are an indication of nutrient deficiency and should be fulfilled in order to meet those requirements. Cravings are natural during pregnancy, however they are not always associated with specific vitamin deficits. It's critical to listen to your body while also making healthy decisions to ensure you achieve your dietary requirements.

7. Herbal Supplements: Some women feel that using herbal supplements or natural therapies during pregnancy is safe. However, many herbs and supplements can be detrimental to a developing infant and should be avoided unless expressly prescribed by a healthcare provider.

Pregnant women should seek advice from healthcare practitioners or registered dietitians if they have any questions or concerns regarding prenatal nutrition, and to ensure they are eating a well-balanced diet that fulfills their particular needs and promotes pregnancy health.

Maternal Nutrition and Fetal Development

Maternal nutrition plays a crucial role in fetal development, as the nutrients provided to the developing baby during pregnancy have a direct impact on its growth, health, and future well-being. Here are a few significant ways that maternal nutrition influences fetal development:

1. Essential Nutrients: Adequate intake of essential nutrients such as folic acid, iron, calcium, protein, omega-3 fatty acids, and vitamins A, C, D, and E is vital for supporting the rapid growth and development of the fetus. These nutrients are involved in various processes such as cell division, organ formation, brain development, and immune function.

2. Brain Development: Nutrients like omega-3 fatty acids (especially DHA) are critical for fetal brain development. DHA is a major component of the brain and retina, and adequate intake during pregnancy is associated with improved cognitive function, vision, and behavior in children.

3. Bone Development: Calcium and vitamin D are essential for the development of strong bones and teeth in the fetus. Insufficient intake of these nutrients during pregnancy can lead to poor bone mineralization in the baby and increase the risk of conditions like rickets.

4. Prevention of Birth Defects: Folic acid is crucial for preventing neural tube defects like spina bifida and anencephaly. Adequate folic acid intake before conception and during early pregnancy is recommended to reduce the risk of these serious birth defects.

5. Immune System Development: Nutrients like vitamin C, vitamin E, zinc, and selenium play a role in supporting the developing immune system of the fetus. A well-nourished mother is more likely to have a baby with a healthy immune system that can fight off infections and diseases.

6. Growth and Birth Weight: Maternal nutrition directly impacts the growth and birth weight of the baby. Inadequate or excessive nutrient intake during pregnancy can lead to low birth weight or macrosomia (high birth weight), both of which are associated with increased risks of health complications for the baby.

7. Long-Term Health: The effects of maternal nutrition on fetal development can have long-lasting implications for the child's health later in life. Poor maternal nutrition during pregnancy has been linked to an increased risk of chronic conditions such as obesity, diabetes, cardiovascular disease, and cognitive impairments in offspring.

It is essential for pregnant women to follow a balanced and nutrient-rich diet, stay hydrated, and avoid harmful substances like alcohol, tobacco, and certain medications to support optimal fetal development. Consulting with healthcare providers or registered dietitians can help ensure that pregnant women are meeting their individual nutritional needs and supporting the healthy growth and development of their babies.

The role of prenatal nutrition in preventing birth defects

Prenatal nutrition plays a crucial role in preventing birth defects, particularly neural tube defects (NTDs) like spina bifida and anencephaly. These serious and often life-threatening birth defects occur when the neural tube, which eventually forms the brain and spinal cord, fails to close properly during early fetal development. Here are some key ways in which prenatal nutrition can help prevent birth defects:

1. **Folic Acid Supplementation**: Folic acid, a B vitamin, is essential for proper neural tube closure and development. Adequate folic acid intake before conception and during the early weeks of pregnancy has been shown to significantly reduce the risk of NTDs. The Centers for Disease Control and Prevention (CDC) recommends that all women of childbearing age consume 400 micrograms of folic acid daily from fortified foods, supplements, or a combination of both.

2. **Fortified Foods and Supplements**: In addition to a healthy diet rich in folate-containing foods like leafy green vegetables, legumes, and citrus fruits, many women may benefit from taking a prenatal vitamin supplement that includes folic acid. This can help ensure that they are getting enough of this crucial nutrient to support proper fetal development.

3. **Early Prenatal Care**: Early initiation of prenatal care is important for identifying any potential nutritional deficiencies or risk factors for birth defects. Healthcare providers can assess a woman's nutritional status, recommend appropriate supplements, and provide guidance on maintaining a healthy diet throughout pregnancy.

4. **Balanced Diet**: In addition to folic acid, other nutrients like iron, calcium, vitamin D, and omega-3 fatty acids are important for supporting overall fetal development and reducing the risk of birth defects. A balanced diet that includes a variety of nutrient-dense foods can help ensure that pregnant women are meeting their nutritional needs.

5. **Avoidance of Harmful Substances**: In addition to ensuring adequate intake of essential nutrients, pregnant women should avoid harmful substances that can increase the risk of birth defects. This includes alcohol, tobacco, certain medications, and exposure to environmental toxins like lead and mercury.

6. **Genetic Counseling**: In cases where there is a family history of birth defects or genetic conditions, genetic counseling may be recommended to assess the risk and provide guidance on prenatal screening and testing options.

By focusing on proper nutrition, supplementation, early prenatal care, and lifestyle choices, women can significantly reduce the risk of birth defects in their babies. It is important for expectant mothers to work closely with healthcare providers to develop a personalized prenatal nutrition plan that supports optimal fetal development and helps prevent birth defects.

CHAPTER 2: NUTRIENT NEEDS DURING PREGNANCY

Essential nutrients for a healthy pregnancy

During pregnancy, the body's nutritional requirements rise to support the fetus' growth and development. A healthy pregnancy and proper fetal growth require a sufficient intake of critical nutrients. Here are some essential nutrients that play an important function during pregnancy:

1. Folic Acid: As previously stated, folic acid is necessary for preventing neural tube abnormalities in the growing baby. It also promotes DNA synthesis and cell division. In addition to fortified meals and pills, folate can be found in leafy green vegetables, lentils, citrus fruits, and fortified cereals.

2. Iron: Iron is required for the formation of red blood cells, which provide oxygen to both the mother and the fetus. Iron deficiency during pregnancy can cause anemia and raise the risk of premature delivery and low birth weight. Lean meats, chicken, fish, beans, and fortified grains are excellent sources of iron.

3. Calcium: Calcium is necessary for the formation of the baby's bones and teeth. It also affects muscular function and nerve transmission. Dairy products, leafy green vegetables, nuts, and fortified foods are high in calcium.

4. **Vitamin D:** Vitamin D promotes bone health and immunological function. It aids the body's absorption of calcium and phosphorus, both of which are necessary for bone formation. Vitamin D sources include sunlight, fatty fish, fortified dairy products, and supplements.

5. **Omega-3 Fatty Acids**: Omega-3 fatty acids, particularly DHA (docosahexaenoic acid), are important for brain and eye development in the fetus. Sources of omega-3 fatty acids include flaxseeds, walnuts fatty fish (such as salmon and sardines), and fortified foods.

6. Protein: Protein is required for tissue growth and repair in both mothers and babies. Lean meats, poultry, fish, eggs, dairy products, legumes, nuts, and seeds are all excellent protein sources.

7. Vitamin A: Vitamin A is essential for vision, immunological function, and cellular development. However, an excessive intake of vitamin A can be detrimental during pregnancy. Sweet potatoes, carrots, spinach, and dairy products are excellent sources of vitamin A.

8. Vitamin C: Vitamin C promotes collagen synthesis, wound healing, and iron absorption. It also functions as an antioxidant, protecting cells from harm. Citrus fruits, strawberries, bell peppers, and broccoli are great sources of vitamin C.

9. Zinc: Zinc is required for immunological function, DNA synthesis, and cellular division. It also influences taste perception and wound healing. Zinc-rich foods include lean meat, poultry, shellfish, whole grains, nuts, and seeds.

10. Iodine: Iodine is essential for thyroid function and brain development in the fetus. Iodized salt, shellfish, dairy products, and seaweed are excellent sources of iodine.

In addition to these critical nutrients, pregnant women should stay hydrated by drinking plenty of water every day. A well-balanced diet rich in nutrient-dense foods will help ensure that both mother and baby get the nutrients they need for a healthy pregnancy. It is crucial for pregnant women to collaborate with healthcare experts to create a personalized dietary plan that addresses their specific needs during this critical period.

Recommended daily intake of micronutrients during pregnancy

The recommended daily intake of macronutrients (carbohydrates, proteins, and fats) and micronutrients during pregnancy can vary depending on individual factors such as age, weight, activity level, and overall health. However, here are general guidelines for pregnant women:

1. Macronutrients:

   - Carbohydrates: Carbohydrates should make up about 45-65% of total daily calories. Choose complex carbohydrates such as whole grains, fruits, vegetables, and legumes for sustained energy.

   - **Proteins**: Protein needs increase during pregnancy to support the growth and development of the baby.
Aim for approximately 71 grams of protein per day. Good sources include lean meats, poultry, fish, eggs, dairy products, legumes, nuts, and seeds.

   - **Fats**: Healthy fats are important for brain development and hormone production. Fats should account for roughly 20-35% of total daily calories. Choose unsaturated fats from avocados, nuts, seeds, olive oil, and fatty fish.

2. **Micronutrients**:

   - **Folic Acid**: The recommended daily intake of folic acid during pregnancy is 600 micrograms. Sources include fortified foods, leafy green vegetables, legumes, citrus fruits, and supplements.

   - **Iron**: Pregnant women need about 27 milligrams of iron per day to prevent anemia and support fetal growth. Good sources include lean meats, poultry, fish, beans, and fortified cereals.

   - **Calcium**: Aim for about 1000 milligrams of calcium per day to support bone development in the baby. Dairy products, leafy green vegetables, nuts, and fortified foods are good sources.

   - **Vitamin D**: The recommended daily intake of vitamin D during pregnancy is 600 IU (International Units). Sunlight exposure, fatty fish, fortified dairy products, and supplements are all potential sources.

   - **Omega-3 Fatty Acids**: Aim for about 200-300 milligrams of DHA per day to support brain and eye development in the fetus. Sources include fortified foods, flaxseeds, walnuts, and fatty fish.

   - **Vitamin A**: The recommended daily intake of vitamin A during pregnancy is 770 micrograms. Good sources include sweet potato, carrots, spinach, and dairy products.

   - **Vitamin C**: Aim for about 85 milligrams of vitamin C per day to support collagen formation and immune function. Citrus fruits, strawberries, bell peppers, and broccoli are among the options.

- **Zinc**: The recommended daily intake of zinc during pregnancy is about 11 milligrams. Good sources include lean meats, poultry, seafood, whole grains, nuts, and seeds.

- **Iodine**: Pregnant women need about 220 micrograms of iodine per day to support thyroid function and brain development in the fetus. Good sources include iodized salt, seafood, dairy products, and seaweed.

It is important for pregnant women to work with healthcare providers or registered dietitians to determine their individual nutrient needs and develop a personalized nutrition plan that meets those needs during pregnancy.

Important hydration and adequate water intake during pregnancy

Hydration and adequate water intake are crucial during pregnancy as they play a vital role in supporting the health and well-being of both the mother and the developing baby. Here are some key reasons why hydration is important during pregnancy:

1. **Supports Fetal Development**: Water is essential for the development of the placenta, which provides nutrients and oxygen to the growing fetus. Proper hydration helps ensure that the baby receives the necessary nutrients for healthy growth and development.

2. **Prevents Dehydration**: Dehydration can lead to a range of issues such as headaches, constipation, urinary tract infections, and preterm labor. Pregnant women are at a higher risk of dehydration due to increased fluid needs, so it is important to stay well-hydrated to prevent these complications.

3. **Regulates Body Temperature**: Pregnant women have an increased metabolic rate, which can lead to higher body temperature. Adequate hydration helps regulate body temperature and prevent overheating, especially during hot weather or physical activity.

4. **Supports Digestion and Nutrient Absorption**: Water plays a key role in digestion and nutrient absorption. It helps break down food, aids in the absorption of nutrients, and prevents constipation, which is a common issue during pregnancy.

5. **Prevents Urinary Tract Infections (UTIs)**: UTIs are more common during pregnancy due to hormonal changes and increased pressure on the bladder. Drinking plenty of water helps flush out bacteria from the urinary tract and reduces the risk of developing UTIs.

6. **Reduces Swelling and Fluid Retention**: Adequate hydration can help reduce swelling and fluid retention, which are common symptoms of pregnancy, especially in the later stages. Drinking enough water helps maintain fluid balance in the body and reduces the risk of edema.

7. **Promotes Healthy Weight Gain**: Staying hydrated can help prevent excessive weight gain during pregnancy. Drinking water instead of sugary beverages can also help reduce empty calories and support healthy weight management.

8. **Supports Circulation**: Proper hydration is essential for maintaining healthy blood volume and circulation, which is important for delivering nutrients and oxygen to the baby through the placenta.

9. **Prevents Preterm Labor**: Dehydration can trigger contractions and potentially lead to preterm labor. By staying well-hydrated, pregnant women can reduce the risk of premature birth.

10. **Improves Energy Levels**: Fatigue is common during pregnancy, and dehydration can exacerbate feelings of tiredness. Drinking enough water throughout the day can help boost energy levels and combat pregnancy-related fatigue.

To ensure adequate hydration during pregnancy, it is recommended that pregnant women drink about 8-10 cups (64-80 ounces) of water per day, in addition to fluids obtained from foods and other beverages. It is crucial to respond to your body's thirst cues and drink water consistently throughout the day. If you have any concerns about hydration or fluid intake during pregnancy, consult with your healthcare provider for personalized recommendations.

Role of prenatal Vitamins in adequate water intake during pregnancy

Prenatal vitamins play a crucial role in meeting the increased nutrient needs of pregnant women and supporting the health and development of both the mother and the growing baby. Here are some key details about the role of prenatal vitamins in meeting nutrient needs during pregnancy:

1. **Folic Acid (Folate)**: One of the most important nutrients in prenatal vitamins is folic acid, which is essential for preventing neural tube defects in the developing baby. Adequate folic acid intake before and during pregnancy is crucial for proper brain and spinal cord development.

2. **Iron**: Iron is another essential nutrient in prenatal vitamins, as pregnant women need more iron to support the increased production of red blood cells and hemoglobin for both the mother and the baby. Iron deficiency in pregnancy can cause anemia, tiredness, and other issues.

3. **Calcium**: Calcium is important for maintaining strong bones and teeth, as well as supporting muscle function and nerve transmission. Prenatal vitamins often contain calcium to help meet the increased demands of pregnancy and ensure optimal bone health for both the mother and the baby.

4. **Iodine**: Iodine is necessary for thyroid function and plays a critical role in fetal brain development. Prenatal vitamins typically include iodine to support proper thyroid function and prevent developmental issues in the baby.

5. **Vitamin D**: Vitamin D is essential for calcium absorption, bone health, and immune function. Adequate vitamin D intake is important during pregnancy to support bone development in the baby and maintain overall health for both the mother and the baby.

6. **Omega-3 Fatty Acids**: Some prenatal vitamins contain omega-3 fatty acids, such as DHA (docosahexaenoic acid), which are important for brain and eye

development in the fetus. Omega-3 fatty acids also support maternal health and may reduce the risk of preterm birth.

7. **Vitamin B12**: Vitamin B12 is necessary for DNA synthesis, red blood cell production, and nerve function. Prenatal vitamins often include vitamin B12 to prevent deficiency and support healthy development in both the mother and the baby.

8. **Vitamin C**: Vitamin C is an antioxidant that supports immune function, collagen production, and iron absorption. Adequate vitamin C intake during pregnancy can help boost immunity, promote wound healing, and support overall health.

9. **Zinc**: Zinc plays a role in cell growth, immune function, and protein synthesis. Prenatal vitamins may contain zinc to support fetal growth and development, as well as maternal health during pregnancy.

10. **Other Nutrients**: Prenatal vitamins may also include other essential nutrients such as vitamin E, vitamin A, magnesium, and other minerals to help meet the increased nutrient needs of pregnant women and ensure optimal health for both the mother and the baby.

It is important for pregnant women to take prenatal vitamins as recommended by their healthcare provider to help fill any nutrient gaps in their diet and support a healthy pregnancy. Prenatal vitamins should complement a balanced diet rich in fruits, vegetables, whole grains, lean proteins, and dairy products to ensure adequate intake of essential nutrients during pregnancy. If you have specific dietary concerns or medical conditions, consult with your healthcare provider or a registered dietitian for personalized recommendations on prenatal vitamin supplementation.

Sources of key nutrients in a prenatal diet

A well-balanced prenatal diet should include a variety of nutrient-dense foods to ensure that both the mother and the growing baby receive all the essential nutrients needed for a healthy pregnancy. Here are some key nutrients and their food sources that are important to include in a prenatal diet:

1. **Folic Acid (Folate)**:
   - Food sources: Leafy green vegetables (spinach, kale, broccoli), legumes (beans, lentils), citrus fruits (oranges, grapefruits), avocados, fortified grains and cereals.

2. **Iron**:
   - Food sources: Red meat (beef, lamb), poultry (chicken, turkey), fish, beans, lentils, tofu, spinach, fortified cereals, pumpkin seeds.

3. **Calcium**:
   - Food sources: Dairy products (milk, yogurt, cheese), fortified plant-based milk (almond milk, soy milk), leafy green vegetables (collard greens, bok choy), tofu, almonds.

4. **Iodine**:
   - Food sources: Seafood (fish, shrimp, seaweed), dairy products, iodized salt, eggs.

5. **Vitamin D**:
   - Food sources: Fatty fish (salmon, mackerel, sardines), fortified dairy products, fortified plant-based milk, eggs.

6. **Omega-3 Fatty Acids (DHA)**:
   - Food sources: Flaxseeds, chia seeds, Fatty fish (salmon, trout, mackerel), walnuts.

7. **Vitamin B12**:
   - Food sources: Animal products (meat, poultry, fish, eggs, dairy products), fortified plant-based foods (nutritional yeast, fortified cereals).

8. **Vitamin C**:
   - Food sources: Citrus fruits (oranges, grapefruits), strawberries, kiwi, bell peppers, broccoli, tomatoes.

9. **Zinc**:

- Food sources: Meat (beef, pork, lamb), poultry (chicken, turkey), seafood (oysters, crab), beans, nuts (cashews, almonds), seeds (pumpkin seeds).

10. **Other Nutrients**:

- **Vitamin E**: Nuts (almonds, hazelnuts), seeds (sunflower seeds), spinach, broccoli.

- **Vitamin A**: Sweet potatoes, carrots, leafy green vegetables (spinach, kale), eggs.

- **Magnesium**: Magnesium-rich foods include almonds, cashews, pumpkin and sunflower seeds, healthy grains, and legumes.

In addition to these key nutrients, it is important for pregnant women to consume a variety of fruits, vegetables, whole grains, lean proteins, and healthy fats to ensure a well-rounded prenatal diet. It is recommended to consult with a healthcare provider or a registered dietitian to create a personalized meal plan that meets individual nutrient needs during pregnancy. Dietary supplements may be recommended if there are specific nutrient deficiencies or challenges meeting nutrient requirements through food alone.

CHAPTER 3: MEAL PLANNING FOR PREGNANCY

Tips for creating a balanced meal plan during pregnancy

Creating a balanced meal plan during pregnancy is crucial to ensure you are getting all the necessary nutrients for your health and the development of your baby. Here are some detailed tips to help you create a well-balanced meal plan:

1. **Include a Variety of Nutrient-Dense Foods**:

   - Aim to include a wide variety of nutrient-dense foods in your meals. This contains fruits and vegetables, entire grains, lean meats, and healthy fats.Different colored fruits and vegetables provide a range of vitamins and minerals, so try to include a rainbow of produce in your diet.

2. **Focus on Whole Grains**:

   - Choose whole grains such as brown rice, quinoa, whole wheat bread, oats, and barley. Whole grains are rich in fiber, B vitamins, and minerals like iron and magnesium, which are important during pregnancy.

3. **Incorporate Lean Proteins**:

   - Include sources of lean protein in your meals such as poultry, fish, lean cuts of beef or pork, eggs, legumes (beans, lentils), tofu, and low-fat dairy products. Protein is required for the growth and development of your kid.

4. **Prioritize Calcium-Rich Foods**:

   - Calcium is important for the development of your baby's bones and teeth. Include dairy products like milk, yogurt, and cheese, as well as fortified plant-based milk alternatives. Leafy greens like kale and broccoli are also good sources of calcium.

5. **Include Healthy Fats**:

   - Omega-3 fatty acids are essential for your baby's cognitive development. Include sources of healthy fats like chia seeds, fatty fish (salmon, sardines), flaxseeds, avocado and walnuts in your diet.

6. Eat Plenty of Fruits and Vegetables:

   - Aim to incorporate a variety of fruits and vegetables into your meals and snacks. These foods provide essential vitamins, minerals, antioxidants, and fiber that support both your health and your baby's development.

7. Stay Hydrated:

   - Drink plenty of water throughout the day to stay hydrated. Adequate hydration is important for maintaining amniotic fluid levels, supporting digestion, and preventing issues like constipation.

8. Limit Processed Foods and Added Sugars:

   - Minimize your intake of processed foods, sugary snacks, and beverages. Opt for whole foods and healthier snack options like fruits, nuts, seeds, yogurt, or whole grain crackers.

9. Snack Smartly:

   - Include healthy snacks in between meals to keep your energy levels stable. Good snack options include fruit with nut butter, yogurt with granola, vegetable sticks with hummus, or a small handful of nuts.

10. Listen to Your Body:

   - Pay heed to your body's hunger and fullness signals. Eat when you're hungry, and quit when you're satisfied. Pregnancy can bring about changes in appetite, so it's important to listen to what your body needs.

11. Take Prenatal Supplements:

   - In addition to a balanced diet, prenatal supplements may be recommended by your healthcare provider to ensure you are meeting all your nutrient needs during pregnancy. These typically include folic acid, iron, calcium, and omega-3 fatty acids.

12. Consult with a Healthcare Provider or Dietitian:

   - If you have specific dietary concerns or questions about your nutrition during pregnancy, consult with a healthcare provider or a registered dietitian who can provide personalized guidance and recommendations tailored to your individual needs.

By following these detailed tips and focusing on nutrient-dense foods, you can create a balanced meal plan that supports a healthy pregnancy for both you and your baby. Remember that every pregnancy is unique, so it's important to listen to your body and seek professional guidance when needed.

Importance of variety and diversity in food choices during pregnancy
Eating a variety of foods during pregnancy is essential to ensure you and your baby receive all the necessary nutrients for optimal health and development. Here are some detailed reasons why variety and diversity in food choices are important during pregnancy:

1. **Nutrient Adequacy**: Different foods contain different nutrients, so consuming a wide variety of foods helps ensure you are getting a broad spectrum of essential vitamins, minerals, antioxidants, and macronutrients. This is crucial for supporting your baby's growth and development and maintaining your own health during pregnancy.

2. **Optimal Nutrient Intake**: Each food group provides a unique set of nutrients. For example, fruits and vegetables are rich in vitamins, minerals, and fiber, while lean proteins offer essential amino acids for tissue growth and repair. Including a variety of foods in your diet helps you meet your daily nutrient requirements without relying on any single food or food group.

3. **Prevention of Nutrient Deficiencies**: By incorporating a diverse range of foods into your meals, you reduce the risk of developing nutrient deficiencies. Certain nutrients like iron, calcium, folic acid, omega-3 fatty acids, and vitamin D are particularly important during pregnancy, and consuming a variety of foods helps ensure you get an adequate intake of these nutrients.

4. **Enhanced Palatability and Enjoyment**: Eating a wide array of foods can make your meals more interesting and enjoyable. Variety in food choices can help

prevent monotony and boredom with your diet, making it easier to maintain healthy eating habits throughout your pregnancy.

5. **Supports Digestive Health**: Different foods contain varying amounts of fiber, which is important for digestive health and preventing issues like constipation—a common concern during pregnancy. Including a variety of high-fiber foods such as fruits, vegetables, whole grains, and legumes can help keep your digestive system running smoothly.

6. **Exposure to Different Flavors and Textures**: Consuming a diverse range of foods during pregnancy can expose your baby to different flavors through the amniotic fluid, potentially influencing their taste preferences later in life. Introducing a variety of flavors and textures early on may help promote a more varied diet for your child in the future.

7. **Balanced Macronutrient Intake**: Including a mix of carbohydrates, proteins, and fats from various sources helps ensure you are getting a balanced intake of macronutrients. This balance is important for providing energy, supporting growth, and maintaining overall health throughout pregnancy.

8. **Adaptation to Changing Nutritional Needs**: As pregnancy progresses, your nutritional needs may change. Eating a diverse range of foods allows you to adapt to these changing needs by providing flexibility in meeting nutrient requirements as your body and baby's needs evolve.

9. **Reduced Risk of Food Boredom or Aversion**: Pregnancy can bring about changes in taste preferences and cravings. Having a variety of food options available can help prevent food aversions or boredom by offering different flavors and textures to choose from.

Incorporating a wide variety of nutrient-dense foods into your diet during pregnancy is key to promoting optimal health for both you and your baby. By focusing on diversity in food choices, you can ensure you are meeting your nutritional needs, enjoying your meals, and supporting a healthy pregnancy journey.

Meal plans for each trimester

Here are sample meal plans for each trimester of pregnancy, including breakfast, lunch, dinner, and snacks. Please note that these meal plans are general suggestions and may need to be adjusted based on your individual dietary preferences, nutritional needs, and any specific recommendations from your healthcare provider.

First Trimester:
Breakfast:
- Scrambled eggs, spinach, and feta cheese
- Whole grain toast with avocado slices
- Fresh fruit salad (berries, oranges, kiwi)

Lunch:
- Quinoa salad made with chickpeas, roasted veggies, and a lemon-tahini dressing.
- Greek yogurt with honey and nuts
- Carrot sticks with hummus

Dinner:
- Steamed broccoli and quinoa alongside baked fish.
- Cherry tomatoes with a mixed green salad dressed with a balsamic vinaigrette.
- Whole grain dinner roll.

Snacks:
- Apple slices with almond butter.
- Trail mix (nuts, seeds, dried fruit).
- Cottage cheese with pineapple chunks.

Second Trimester:
Breakfast:
- Chia seed overnight oats with almond milk and a variety of berries.
- Whole grain toast with peanut butter
- Green smoothie (spinach, banana, almond milk)

Lunch:
- Turkey and avocado wrap with whole grain tortilla
- Whole grain crackers served alongside lentil soup
- Baby carrots with tzatziki sauce

Dinner:
- Grilled chicken breast served with asparagus and sweet potato wedges

- Quinoa pilaf with roasted vegetables.
- Mixed berry parfait with Greek yogurt.

Snacks:
- Edamame pods
- Rice cakes with hummus and cucumber slices
- Greek yogurt with granola

Third Trimester:

Breakfast:
- Whole grain pancakes with sliced bananas and maple syrup
- Hard-boiled eggs
- Fresh orange juice

Lunch:
- Spinach and strawberry salad with grilled chicken strips and balsamic vinaigrette
- Whole grain pita bread with tzatziki sauce
- Cherry tomatoes with mozzarella cheese

Dinner:
- Beef stir-fry with bell peppers, broccoli, and brown rice
- Mixed green salad with avocado slices and citrus dressing
- Whole grain dinner roll

Snacks:
- Cottage cheese with peach slices
- Almond butter on rice cakes
- Vegetable sticks with guacamole

Remember to stay hydrated throughout the day by drinking plenty of water and listen to your body's hunger cues. It's essential to consult with your healthcare provider or a registered dietitian to ensure you're meeting your specific nutritional needs during each trimester of pregnancy.

Incorporating nutrient dense foods into a prenatal diet

A prenatal diet that supports the health of the mother and the developing baby must include nutrient-dense foods and superfoods. Pregnancy increases nutritional needs, and these foods, being high in vitamins, minerals, antioxidants, and other critical nutrients, can help meet those needs. The following are some superfoods and nutrient-dense foods to think about incorporating into your pregnancy diet:

1. Leafy Greens: Vitamins A, C, K, and folate are abundant in foods including spinach, kale, Swiss chard, and collard greens. They also supply vital minerals, such as calcium and iron, which are necessary for a successful pregnancy.

2. Berries: High in fiber, vitamin C, and antioxidants, berries like blueberries, strawberries, raspberries, and blackberries are highly recommended. Along with supporting digestion and supplying vital nutrients for embryonic growth, they can help strengthen immunity.

3. Legumes: Beans, lentils, chickpeas, and peas are high in plant-based protein, fiber, iron, folate, and other minerals. They can aid to promote healthy growth and development throughout pregnancy.

4. Whole Grains: Quinoa, brown rice, oats, and whole wheat contain complex carbohydrates, fiber, vitamins, and minerals. They can help regulate blood sugar levels, aid digestion, and provide steady energy throughout the day.

5. Fatty Fish: Rich in omega-3 fatty acids, which are crucial for brain development and general health, salmon, mackerel, sardines, and trout are examples of fatty fish. Additionally, during pregnancy, omega-3s can promote cardiovascular health and lessen inflammation.

6. Nuts and Seeds: Rich in protein, fiber, vitamins, and minerals, almonds, walnuts, chia seeds, flaxseeds, and pumpkin seeds are excellent sources of healthy fats. They can lower inflammation, promote brain function, and give mother and child vital nutrients.

7. Dairy Products: Rich in calcium, protein, vitamin D, and other minerals that are critical for bone formation and health are yogurt, cheese, and milk. Limit the amount of saturated fat you consume by choosing low- or no-fat foods.

8. Avocado: Avocado is a nutrient-dense fruit high in healthy fats, fiber, folate, potassium, and vitamins C and E. They can help in fetal growth and development while also providing critical nutrients to the mother.

9. Eggs: Eggs include protein, choline, iron, and other minerals essential for embryonic brain development and overall wellness. Choose organic or pasture-raised eggs for more nutrients.

10. Sweet Potatoes: They are high in beta-carotene, fiber, vitamin C, and potassium. They can improve immunological function, digestion, and supply essential nutrients for a healthy pregnancy.

Your prenatal diet can help make sure you are getting the extra nourishment you need throughout pregnancy by including a range of these nutrient-dense foods and superfoods. It's crucial to speak with a qualified dietician or your healthcare practitioner to develop a customized meal plan that suits your tastes and requirements. During this unique time, keep in mind that you should prioritize a balanced diet that consists of a range of foods to support both your health and your baby's health.

Strategies for managing cravings and aversions while maintaining a healthy diet.

Managing cravings and aversions while maintaining a healthy diet during pregnancy can be challenging, but it is possible with some strategies. The following advice will assist you in navigating these changes:

1. **Listen to Your Body:** Pay attention to your body's signals and cravings. Cravings can sometimes be your body's way of signaling a need for specific nutrients. Try to identify if there is a pattern to your cravings and choose healthier options that fulfill those needs.

2. **Plan Ahead:** Stock your kitchen with healthy snacks and meal options that are in line with your nutritional needs. Having nutritious foods readily available can help you make better choices when cravings strike.

3. **Balance Your Meals:** Aim for balanced meals that include a mix of protein, healthy fats, complex carbohydrates, and fiber. This can help stabilize blood sugar levels and reduce the likelihood of intense cravings.

4. **Include Variety:** Incorporate a variety of foods in your diet to ensure you are getting a wide range of nutrients. This can also help prevent boredom with your meals and reduce the chances of developing strong cravings for specific foods.

5. **Stay Hydrated:** Sometimes thirst can be mistaken for hunger or cravings. Stay hydrated throughout the day by drinking lots of water, which can also help you resist unneeded cravings.

6. **Healthy Substitutions:** If you are craving something sweet, try reaching for fresh fruit or a small piece of dark chocolate instead of sugary snacks. If you are craving salty foods, opt for roasted nuts or whole grain crackers with hummus.

7. **Mindful Eating:** Practice mindful eating by paying attention to your hunger and fullness cues. Eat slowly, savor each bite, and stop when you feel satisfied rather than overly full.

8. **Stay Active:** Regular physical activity can help manage cravings and boost your mood. Engage in activities that you enjoy, such as walking, prenatal yoga, or swimming, to help distract yourself from cravings.

9. **Seek Support:** Talk to your healthcare provider or a registered dietitian if you are struggling with intense cravings or aversions that are impacting your ability to maintain a healthy diet. They are able to offer tailored advice and assistance.

10. **Indulge in Moderation:** It's okay to indulge in your cravings occasionally, as long as it's done in moderation and balanced with nutrient-dense foods. You deserve to feel free to indulge in a tiny bit of your favorite treat.

Remember that pregnancy is a unique time when your body's needs may change, so it's important to be flexible and kind to yourself as you navigate cravings and aversions while maintaining a healthy diet.

CHAPTER 4: FOOD SAFETY DURING PREGNANCY.

Safe food handling and preparation during pregnancy

Safe food handling and preparation are crucial during pregnancy to prevent foodborne illnesses that can harm both the mother and the developing baby. Here are some guidelines for safe food handling and preparation during pregnancy:

1. **Wash Hands**: Always wash your hands with soap and water before handling food, especially after touching raw meat, poultry, seafood, or eggs.

2. **Separate Raw and Cooked Foods**: Keep raw meats, poultry, seafood, and eggs separate from ready-to-eat foods to avoid cross-contamination. Use different cutting boards and cutlery for raw and cooked meals.

3. **Cook Thoroughly**: Cook all meats, poultry, seafood, and eggs thoroughly to kill harmful bacteria. Use a food thermometer to ensure that these foods reach the recommended internal temperature:

   - Beef, pork, lamb: 145°F (63°C)
   - Ground meat: 160°F (71°C)
   - Poultry: 165°F (74°C)
   - Seafood: 145°F (63°C)

4. **Avoid Raw or Undercooked Foods**: Avoid consuming raw or undercooked meats, poultry, seafood, and eggs, as they may contain harmful bacteria such as Salmonella, Listeria, and E. coli.

5. **Handle Produce Safely**: Wash fruits and vegetables thoroughly under running water before eating or cooking them. Use a produce brush for firm produce like melons or cucumbers.

6. **Refrigerate Properly**: Refrigerate perishable foods promptly to prevent bacterial growth. Keep the refrigerator temperature at 40°F (4°C) or below and the freezer at 0°F (-18°C) or below.

7. **Use Safe Water**: Drink and use only safe water for cooking and drinking. If you are concerned about the safety of your tap water, try using bottled or filtered water.

8. **Avoid High-Risk Foods**: Avoid high-risk foods that are more likely to cause foodborne illnesses, such as unpasteurized dairy products, raw sprouts, deli meats, and refrigerated pâté or meat spreads.

9. **Be Mindful of Mercury**: Limit consumption of fish high in mercury, such as shark, swordfish, king mackerel, and tilefish. Choose fish lower in mercury, like salmon, shrimp, pollock, and catfish.

10. **Follow Food Safety Guidelines**: Follow food safety guidelines when eating out or ordering takeout. Ensure that restaurants follow proper food handling practices to reduce the risk of foodborne illnesses.

By following these guidelines for safe food handling and preparation during pregnancy, you can reduce the risk of foodborne illnesses and protect both yourself and your baby. If you have any concerns or questions about food safety during pregnancy, consult with your healthcare provider or a registered dietitian for personalized advice.

Common foodborne illnesses to be aware of during pregnancy

During pregnancy, it is critical to be aware of frequent foodborne infections that can harm both the mother and the growing baby. Here are some of the most frequent foodborne illnesses to be aware of while pregnant:

1. **Listeriosis**: What causes listeriosis is a bacterium called Listeria monocytogenes. Owing to immunological system alterations, pregnant women are more susceptible to listeriosis. The major side effects of listeriosis might include miscarriage, stillbirth, early birth, or serious disease in infants. There could be symptoms including diarrhea, soreness in the muscles, nausea, and fever. Deli meats, hot dogs, chilled smoked seafood, and unpasteurized dairy products are among the foods that are commonly connected to Listeria disease.

2. **Toxoplasmosis**: The parasite Toxoplasma is the cause of toxoplasmosis. If a pregnant woman gets toxoplasmosis, the infection can transfer to the fetus and cause major health issues. Muscle aches, enlarged lymph nodes, and flu-like symptoms are some of the signs and symptoms of toxoplasmosis. Raw or undercooked meat, unclean fruits and vegetables, tainted water, and cat excrement can all contain Toxoplasma.

3. **Salmonellosis**: It is the Salmonella bacteria that cause salmonellosis. Severe diarrhea, fever, cramping in the abdomen, and vomiting are some of the signs and symptoms of salmonellosis among expectant mothers. Poultry, meat, eggs, raw or undercooked meat, unpasteurized dairy products, and contaminated fruit can all harbor Salmonella, which can cause dehydration and premature birth.

4. **Campylobacteriosis**: Campylobacteriosis is caused by the Campylobacter bacteria. Campylobacteriosis symptoms include diarrhea (usually bloody), stomach cramps, fever, and nausea. Severe Campylobacter infection during pregnancy might result in problems such as miscarriage or preterm birth. Campylobacter can be found in undercooked poultry, unpasteurized milk, and polluted water.

5. **E. coli Infection**: Foodborne disease can be caused by specific strains of Escherichia coli (E. coli). Vomiting, severe stomach cramps, and diarrhea—often bloody—are signs of an E. coli infection. An E. Coli infection during pregnancy can cause major side effects such hemolytic uremic syndrome (HUS), which can cause renal failure. Raw fruits and vegetables, unpasteurized dairy products, undercooked ground beef, and tainted water can all contain E. coli.

6. **Norovirus**:The virus that causes gastroenteritis is extremely contagious. Frequent signs of a norovirus infection include fever, cramping in the stomach, vomiting, and diarrhea. Restaurants and cruise ships are examples of places where norovirus outbreaks can happen where food is produced or served.

Pregnant women must take steps to avoid foodborne diseases by using safe food handling procedures, avoiding high-risk foods, and ensuring proper cooking and storage of food. If you suspect you have contracted a foodborne illness while pregnant, get medical attention right away to receive proper treatment and preserve the health of both you and your baby.

Potential risks associated with certain foods.

Certain foods can pose risks during pregnancy due to their potential to cause foodborne illnesses, harm the developing fetus, or lead to complications. Here are detailed explanations of the potential risks associated with specific foods during pregnancy:

1. Raw or Undercooked Meat, Poultry, and Seafood:
- These foods may contain harmful bacteria like Salmonella, E. coli, or Listeria, which can cause foodborne illnesses such as food poisoning.
- Infections from these bacteria can lead to symptoms like nausea, vomiting, diarrhea, and fever, which can be particularly dangerous during pregnancy.
- Some bacteria, like Listeria, can cross the placenta and infect the fetus, leading to miscarriage, preterm birth, or serious health issues for the baby.

2. Unpasteurized Dairy Products:
- Raw milk and cheeses made from unpasteurized milk can harbor harmful bacteria like Listeria, E. coli, or Salmonella.
- Pregnancy-related listeria infection can raise the risk of stillbirth, early delivery, miscarriage, and potentially fatal illnesses in the unborn child.

- Pasteurization is a process that kills harmful bacteria without affecting the nutritional value of dairy products, making pasteurized options safer for pregnant women.

3. Raw Eggs:
- Raw or undercooked eggs may contain Salmonella bacteria, which can cause severe food poisoning.
- Infections with Salmonella can lead to symptoms like abdominal pain, diarrhea, fever, and dehydration, posing risks to both the mother and the developing fetus.

- Cooking eggs thoroughly until the yolks and whites are firm can help eliminate the risk of Salmonella contamination.

4. Deli Meats and Hot Dogs:
- Processed meats like deli meats and hot dogs may be contaminated with Listeria bacteria during processing or storage.
- Listeria infection can cause flu-like symptoms in pregnant women but may lead to severe complications in the fetus, including miscarriage, stillbirth, or serious health issues.
- Heating deli meats and hot dogs until they are steaming hot can help reduce the risk of Listeria contamination.

5. High-Mercury Fish:
- Certain fish species like shark, swordfish, king mackerel, and tilefish contain high levels of mercury, a toxic metal that can harm the nervous system of the developing fetus.
- Mercury exposure during pregnancy has been linked to developmental delays, cognitive impairments, and other neurological issues in children.
- Pregnant women are advised to limit consumption of high-mercury fish and opt for lower-mercury alternatives like salmon, shrimp, or canned light tuna.

6. Excess Caffeine:
- High levels of caffeine consumption during pregnancy have been associated with an increased risk of miscarriage, preterm birth, low birth weight, and other complications.
- Caffeine crosses the placenta and reaches the fetus, potentially affecting their heart rate and metabolism.
- Limiting caffeine intake to less than 200 milligrams per day (equivalent to about one 12-ounce cup of coffee) is recommended to minimize potential risks.

7. Alcohol:
- Alcohol consumption during pregnancy can lead to a range of birth defects and developmental issues collectively known as Fetal Alcohol Spectrum Disorders (FASDs).

- Alcohol crosses the placenta and can interfere with fetal development, causing physical abnormalities, cognitive impairments, behavioral problems, and lifelong disabilities.
- The safest approach is to abstain from alcohol completely during pregnancy to protect the health and well-being of both the mother and the baby.

8. Unwashed Fruits and Vegetables:
- Fruits and vegetables that are not properly washed may carry contaminants like pesticides, soil residues, or harmful bacteria.
- Ingesting these contaminants can increase the risk of foodborne illnesses or exposure to toxic substances during pregnancy.
- Thoroughly washing fruits and vegetables under running water before consumption can help remove potential hazards and reduce the risk of foodborne infections.

9. Raw Sprouts:
- Raw sprouts like alfalfa, clover, and radish are prone to bacterial contamination during growth and harvesting.
- Sprouts have been linked to outbreaks of foodborne illnesses caused by pathogens like E. coli or Salmonella.
- Pregnant women should avoid consuming raw sprouts or opt for cooked varieties to minimize the risk of bacterial infections.

10. Excessively Salty or Sugary Foods:
- Consuming foods high in salt or sugar during pregnancy can contribute to health issues like high blood pressure, gestational diabetes, excessive weight gain, and other complications.
- Excessive salt intake can lead to fluid retention and increased blood pressure, potentially affecting maternal and fetal health.
- High sugar consumption may raise the risk of gestational diabetes, which can have adverse effects on pregnancy outcomes and increase the likelihood of future health problems for both mother and child.

By being aware of these potential risks associated with certain foods during pregnancy and making informed dietary choices, pregnant women can help safeguard their health and promote a healthy pregnancy for themselves and their babies. It is essential to consult with healthcare providers for personalized guidance on nutrition and dietary restrictions during pregnancy.

List of foods to avoid or limit during pregnancy.

During pregnancy, it is important to be cautious about the foods you consume to ensure the health and safety of both you and your baby. Here is a comprehensive list of foods to avoid or limit during pregnancy:

1. Raw or undercooked meat, poultry, and seafood: These may contain harmful bacteria or parasites that can cause foodborne illnesses.

2. Unpasteurized dairy products: Raw milk and cheeses made from unpasteurized milk can contain harmful bacteria like listeria, which can lead to serious complications during pregnancy.

3. Raw eggs: Avoid consuming raw or undercooked eggs as they may contain salmonella bacteria.

4. Deli meats and hot dogs: These may be contaminated with listeria bacteria, which can be harmful during pregnancy.

5. High-mercury fish: Limit consumption of high-mercury fish such as shark, swordfish, king mackerel, and tilefish, as mercury can harm the developing nervous system of the fetus.

6. Excess caffeine: Limit your intake of caffeine to less than 200 milligrams per day, as high levels of caffeine have been linked to an increased risk of miscarriage and low birth weight.

7. Alcohol: It is recommended to avoid alcohol completely during pregnancy as it can harm the developing fetus and lead to a range of birth defects.

8. Unwashed fruits and vegetables: Make sure to thoroughly wash all fruits and vegetables to remove any potential contaminants like pesticides or bacteria.

9. Raw sprouts: Avoid consuming raw sprouts such as alfalfa, clover, and radish as they may be contaminated with harmful bacteria like E. coli or salmonella.

10. Excessively salty or sugary foods: Limit your intake of foods high in salt or sugar, as excessive consumption can lead to health issues like high blood pressure or gestational diabetes.

It is important to consult with your healthcare provider for personalized dietary recommendations during pregnancy.

Alternatives and substitutes for restricted foods
To ensure that pregnant women receive essential nutrients while avoiding potentially risky foods, here are some alternatives and substitutions that can help meet nutritional needs:

1. Protein:
- Instead of raw or undercooked meat, poultry, and seafood, opt for cooked lean meats like chicken, turkey, or beef.
- Choose well-cooked fish low in mercury, such as salmon, trout, or sardines.
- Incorporate plant-based protein sources like beans, lentils, tofu, and nuts into meals.

2. Calcium:
- Substitute unpasteurized dairy products with pasteurized options like milk, cheese, and yogurt.
- Include calcium-rich foods like fortified plant-based milk, dark leafy greens (e.g., kale, spinach), and almonds in the diet.

3. Iron:
- Consume iron-rich foods such as cooked lean meats, poultry, beans, lentils, and fortified cereals.
- To improve iron absorption, combine foods high in iron with foods high in vitamin C, such as citrus fruits, bell peppers, or strawberries.

4. Folate:
- Choose folate-rich foods like leafy greens, citrus fruits, avocados, and fortified cereals.
- Consider taking a prenatal vitamin containing folic acid to meet increased folate requirements during pregnancy.

5. Omega-3 Fatty Acids:
- Include sources of omega-3 fatty acids like flaxseeds, chia seeds, walnuts, and algae-based supplements in the diet.
- Consume fatty fish low in mercury such as salmon, anchovies, or herring to support brain and eye development in the fetus.

6. Fiber:
- Choose whole grains over refined grains, such as quinoa, brown rice, oats, and whole wheat bread.
- Include fiber-rich fruits and vegetables such as berries, apples, broccoli, and sweet potatoes in meals and snacks.

7. Vitamin D:
- Seek sunlight exposure or consider a vitamin D supplement recommended by a healthcare provider to support bone health and immune function.
- Include vitamin D-fortified foods like fortified milk, orange juice, or cereals in the diet.

8. Vitamin C:
- Incorporate vitamin C-rich fruits and vegetables such as oranges, kiwi, bell peppers, and tomatoes to support immune function and iron absorption.
- Avoid excessive intake of vitamin C supplements and focus on obtaining nutrients from whole foods.

9. Magnesium:
- Include magnesium-rich foods like nuts, seeds, whole grains, leafy greens, and legumes in the diet to support muscle function and energy production.
- Consider magnesium supplements under the guidance of a healthcare provider if dietary intake is insufficient.

10. Antioxidants:
- Consume a variety of colorful fruits and vegetables to obtain antioxidants that help protect cells from damage and support overall health.
- Include berries, dark leafy greens, sweet potatoes, and bell peppers in meals to boost antioxidant intake.

By incorporating these nutrient-rich alternatives into their diet plans and consulting with healthcare providers for personalized recommendations, pregnant women can maintain a balanced and nourishing eating pattern that supports maternal health and fetal development during pregnancy.

Safe food preparation and storage during pregnancy

During pregnancy, it is crucial to follow food safety guidelines to protect both the mother and the developing baby from foodborne illnesses. Here are some key recommendations for safe food preparation and storage during pregnancy:

1. Wash Hands: Always wash your hands thoroughly with soap and water before handling food to prevent the spread of bacteria and viruses.

2. Clean Surfaces: Keep kitchen surfaces, utensils, and cutting boards clean and sanitized to avoid cross-contamination between raw and cooked foods.

3. Separate Raw and Cooked Foods: Store raw meats, poultry, seafood, and eggs away from ready-to-eat foods to prevent the spread of harmful bacteria.

4. Cook Foods Thoroughly: Cook meats, poultry, seafood, and eggs to their recommended internal temperatures to kill any harmful bacteria.

5. Avoid Raw or Undercooked Foods: Avoid consuming raw or undercooked meats, seafood, eggs, and unpasteurized dairy products, as they may contain harmful bacteria such as Listeria, Salmonella, or E. coli.

6. Refrigerate Perishable Foods Promptly: Refrigerate perishable foods, including leftovers, within two hours of cooking to prevent bacterial growth. Keep the refrigerator temperature at or below 40°F (4°C).

7. Use Safe Water Sources: Ensure that the water used for drinking, cooking, and washing fruits and vegetables is safe and free from contaminants.

8. Wash Fruits and Vegetables: Thoroughly wash fruits and vegetables under running water before consuming them to remove dirt, bacteria, and pesticides.

9. Avoid High-Mercury Fish: Limit consumption of high-mercury fish such as shark, swordfish, king mackerel, and tilefish, as mercury exposure can harm the developing baby's nervous system.

10. Check Food Labels: Read food labels carefully to check for expiration dates, storage instructions, and proper handling recommendations to ensure food safety.

11. Be Cautious with Deli Meats and Unpasteurized Products: Avoid consuming deli meats, hot dogs, unpasteurized cheeses, and other products that may contain Listeria bacteria, which can be harmful during pregnancy.

12. Follow Safe Food Handling Practices: Use separate cutting boards for raw meats and produce, avoid cross-contamination, and practice good hygiene when preparing meals to reduce the risk of foodborne illnesses.

By following these guidelines for safe food preparation and storage during pregnancy, expectant mothers can reduce the risk of foodborne infections and promote the health and well-being of themselves and their babies. If you have any specific dietary concerns or questions during pregnancy, consult with a healthcare provider or a registered dietitian for personalized guidance.

CHAPTER 5: MANAGING MORNING SICKNESS AND FOOD AVERSION

Coping with morning sickness

Morning sickness and nausea are common symptoms experienced by many pregnant women, especially during the first trimester. Coping with these symptoms can be challenging, but there are several strategies that may help alleviate discomfort and manage morning sickness effectively. Here are some tips for coping with morning sickness and nausea during pregnancy:

1. Eat Small, Frequent Meals: Instead of large meals, opt for smaller, more frequent meals throughout the day to help prevent an empty stomach, which can trigger nausea.

2. Stay Hydrated: Drink plenty of fluids, such as water, herbal teas, or clear broths, to stay hydrated and prevent dehydration, which can worsen nausea.

3. Avoid Trigger Foods: Identify and avoid foods or smells that trigger your nausea, such as spicy or greasy foods, strong odors, or caffeine.

4. Choose Bland Foods: Opt for bland, easily digestible foods like crackers, toast, rice, bananas, or applesauce that may be easier on your stomach.

5. Ginger: Ginger has natural anti-nausea properties. You can try ginger tea, ginger candies, ginger ale, or ginger supplements to help alleviate nausea.

6. Acupressure Bands: Some women find relief from morning sickness by wearing acupressure bands on their wrists, which apply pressure to specific points that may help reduce nausea.

7. Get Fresh Air: Open windows or go outside for fresh air to help alleviate feelings of nausea and improve overall well-being.

8. Rest and Relaxation: Fatigue and stress can worsen nausea. Make sure to get plenty of rest and practice relaxation techniques such as deep breathing or meditation.

9. Avoid Strong Smells: Strong odors can trigger nausea. Try to stay away from cooking smells, perfumes, or other scents that may exacerbate your symptoms.

10. Vitamin B6 Supplements: Some women find relief from morning sickness by taking vitamin B6 supplements under the guidance of their healthcare provider.

11. Consult Your Healthcare Provider: If your morning sickness is severe and persistent, or if you are unable to keep any food or fluids down, consult your healthcare provider for further evaluation and possible treatment options.

Keep in mind that every woman has a different experience with morning sickness, so what works for one may not work for another. It's essential to listen to your body, experiment with different coping strategies, and seek support from your healthcare provider if you need additional help managing your symptoms.

Nutrient-dense foods good for the body

Nutrient-dense foods that are gentle on the stomach and easy to digest can be beneficial for individuals experiencing digestive issues, including morning sickness during pregnancy or other gastrointestinal discomfort. These foods are typically well-tolerated and provide essential nutrients that can support overall health and well-being. Here are some examples of nutrient-dense foods that are gentle on the stomach and easy to digest:

1. Bananas: Bananas are a great source of potassium, fiber, and vitamin C. They can help calm an upset stomach and are simple to digest.

2. Rice: White rice is a bland, low-fiber food that is gentle on the stomach and easy to digest. It can be a good option for settling an upset stomach or providing energy during times of digestive discomfort.

3. Applesauce: Applesauce is a soft, easily digestible food that can provide fiber, vitamins, and minerals. It is often well-tolerated by individuals with sensitive stomachs.

4. Oatmeal: Oatmeal is a nutritious whole grain that is rich in fiber and provides sustained energy. It is gentle on the stomach and can be a comforting option for breakfast or snacks.

5. Boiled or Steamed Vegetables: Cooked vegetables such as carrots, zucchini, and sweet potatoes are easier to digest than raw vegetables. They provide essential vitamins, minerals, and fiber while being gentle on the stomach.

6. Lean Protein: Lean protein sources like chicken, turkey, fish, or tofu can be easier to digest than fatty or heavily processed meats. They provide essential amino acids for muscle health and overall well-being.

7. Yogurt: Plain, unsweetened yogurt contains probiotics that can support digestive health by promoting the growth of beneficial gut bacteria. It is a good source of protein, calcium, and other nutrients that are gentle on the stomach.

8. Bone Broth: Bone broth is rich in nutrients like collagen, gelatin, and amino acids that can support gut health and digestion. It is soothing to the stomach and can be beneficial during times of digestive distress.

9. Herbal Teas: Chamomile, ginger, peppermint, or fennel tea are known for their calming and digestive properties. These herbal teas can help soothe an upset stomach and promote healthy digestion.

10. Nut Butters: Natural nut butters like almond or cashew butter provide healthy fats, protein, and fiber in a form that is easy to digest. They can be spread on toast or crackers for a nutritious snack.

When choosing nutrient-dense foods that are gentle on the stomach and easy to digest, it's essential to listen to your body's cues and choose foods that make you feel comfortable and nourished. Experiment with different options to find what works best for you and consult with a healthcare provider or dietitian if you have specific dietary concerns or restrictions.

Tips for staying hydrated and maintaining adequate food nutrition

Staying hydrated and maintaining adequate nutrition despite food aversions can be challenging, especially during pregnancy or when experiencing digestive issues. The following advice will help you maintain your nutrition and hydration:

1. Drink Plenty of Water: Hydration is essential for overall health and well-being. Aim to drink at least 8-10 cups of water or more per day, if you are pregnant or breastfeeding. If plain water is unappealing, try adding a splash of fruit juice or infusing it with fresh fruits like lemon or cucumber for flavor.

2. Try Hydrating Foods: In addition to drinking water, include hydrating foods in your diet such as water-rich fruits and vegetables like watermelon, cucumber, oranges, and strawberries. These foods can help you stay hydrated and provide essential vitamins and minerals.

3. Opt for Small, Frequent Meals: If you have food aversions or difficulty eating large meals, try eating smaller, more frequent meals throughout the day. This can help you get the nutrients you need without feeling overwhelmed by a big meal.

4. Focus on Nutrient-Dense Foods: Choose nutrient-dense foods that are rich in vitamins, minerals, and other essential nutrients to support your health.Eat a diet rich in whole grains, lean meats, fruits, veggies, and healthy fats.

5. Experiment with Different Foods: If certain foods trigger aversions or are difficult to digest, try experimenting with different foods to find what works best for you. Be open to trying new foods or preparing familiar foods in different ways to make them more appealing.

6. Consider Liquid or Soft Foods: If solid foods are challenging to eat, consider incorporating liquid or soft foods into your diet such as smoothies, soups, yogurt, or pureed fruits and vegetables. These options can be easier to digest and may be more tolerable if you have food aversions.

7. Take Prenatal Vitamins: If you are unable to meet your nutrient needs through diet alone, consider taking prenatal vitamins to ensure you are getting essential vitamins and minerals, especially during pregnancy or times of increased nutrient requirements.

8. Listen to Your Body: Pay attention to your body's cues and honor your cravings and aversions as much as possible. If a particular food doesn't sit well with you, try to find alternative options that provide similar nutrients.

9. Seek Support from a Healthcare Provider or Dietitian: If you are struggling to stay hydrated and maintain adequate nutrition due to food aversions or other challenges, consider seeking guidance from a healthcare provider or registered dietitian. They can provide personalized recommendations and support to help you meet your nutritional needs.

By incorporating these tips into your daily routine, you can stay hydrated and nourished despite food aversions or digestive issues. Remember to be patient with yourself and prioritize your health and well-being during this time.

Herbal remedies and natural solutions for managing morning sickness.
Morning sickness, or nausea and vomiting during pregnancy, can be a common and challenging symptom for many pregnant individuals. While severe cases may require medical intervention, there are several herbal remedies and natural solutions that may help manage mild to moderate morning sickness. It's important to consult with a healthcare provider before using any herbal remedies, especially during pregnancy, to ensure they are safe and appropriate for your individual situation.

1. Ginger: Ginger is a well-known natural remedy for nausea and has been used for centuries to alleviate digestive issues. You can consume ginger in various forms, such as ginger tea, ginger ale, ginger candies, or ginger supplements. Some studies suggest that ginger may help reduce nausea and vomiting associated with pregnancy.

2. Peppermint: Peppermint is another herb that is known for its calming effect on the digestive system. Peppermint tea or peppermint essential oil may help alleviate nausea and soothe an upset stomach. Be cautious with peppermint oil during pregnancy, as high doses may not be safe.

3. Lemon: The scent of fresh lemon or lemon essential oil may help reduce nausea and improve overall digestion. Sipping on warm lemon water or inhaling the aroma of lemon essential oil may provide relief from morning sickness.

4. Chamomile: Chamomile tea is known for its calming properties and may help ease nausea and promote relaxation. Drinking chamomile tea throughout the day or before bedtime may help manage morning sickness symptoms.

5. Acupressure: Acupressure wristbands, which apply pressure to specific points on the wrist, have been shown to help alleviate nausea and vomiting. These wristbands can be worn throughout the day and may provide relief from morning sickness symptoms.

6. Vitamin B6: Vitamin B6 (pyridoxine) is a nutrient that has been studied for its potential to reduce nausea and vomiting during pregnancy. Consult with your healthcare provider about the appropriate dosage of vitamin B6 for managing morning sickness.

7. Small, Frequent Meals: Eating small, frequent meals throughout the day can help stabilize blood sugar levels and prevent feelings of nausea. Avoiding large meals or long periods without eating may help manage morning sickness symptoms.

8. Stay Hydrated: Dehydration can worsen nausea, so it's important to stay hydrated by sipping on water, herbal teas, or electrolyte-rich beverages throughout the day.

9. Rest and Relaxation: Stress and fatigue can exacerbate morning sickness symptoms, so prioritizing rest and relaxation can be beneficial. Practice relaxation

techniques such as deep breathing, meditation, or gentle yoga to help manage stress and promote overall well-being.

It's essential to listen to your body and find what works best for you when managing morning sickness naturally. If your symptoms are severe or persistent, consult with your healthcare provider for personalized recommendations and guidance on managing morning sickness during pregnancy.

CHAPTER 6: GESTATIONAL DIABETES AND PRENATAL NUTRITION.

Gestational diabetes and its Effect on pregnancy

Gestational diabetes is a kind of diabetes that occurs during pregnancy and usually goes away after childbirth. It is distinguished by high blood sugar levels, which can be dangerous to both the mother and the infant. The condition occurs when the body cannot produce enough insulin to meet the increased demands of pregnancy.

Overview of Gestational Diabetes and Its Effects on Pregnancy:

1. Diagnosis: Gestational diabetes is usually diagnosed between the 24th and 28th week of pregnancy through a glucose tolerance test. Some women may have risk factors that require earlier screening.

2. Impact on Mother:
   - Increased Risk of Type 2 Diabetes: Women with gestational diabetes have a higher risk of developing type 2 diabetes later in life.
   - Pregnancy Complications: Gestational diabetes can lead to complications such as preeclampsia, cesarean delivery, and preterm birth.
   - Increased Risk of Future Pregnancies: Women who have had gestational diabetes are at a higher risk of developing the condition in subsequent pregnancies.

3. Impact on Baby:
   - Macrosomia: Babies born to mothers with gestational diabetes may be larger than average (macrosomia), increasing the risk of birth injuries.

- Hypoglycemia: Infants born to mothers with gestational diabetes may experience low blood sugar levels (hypoglycemia) after birth.

- Respiratory Distress Syndrome: Babies born to mothers with gestational diabetes are at a higher risk of respiratory distress syndrome.

4. Management:

- Blood Sugar Monitoring: Women with gestational diabetes need to monitor their blood sugar levels regularly to ensure they are within target ranges.

- Diet and Exercise: A well-balanced diet and regular exercise can help control blood sugar levels and reduce the risk of complications.

- Medication: In some circumstances, insulin or oral medicines may be required to maintain blood sugar levels.

5. Follow-Up Care:

-Postpartum Screening: Women who have gestational diabetes should have their blood sugar levels checked after giving birth.

- Lifestyle Changes: Maintaining a healthy weight and remaining physically active can help prevent or delay the onset of type 2 diabetes.

To sum up, gestational diabetes during pregnancy can have serious consequences for both the mother and the unborn child. To lower the condition's dangers and guarantee a successful pregnancy, early detection, appropriate treatment, and aftercare are crucial. When a pregnant person has gestational diabetes, it's critical that they collaborate closely with their medical professionals to monitor their condition and make decisions about their care.

Managing gestational diabetes

Dietary management plays a crucial role in the management of gestational diabetes by helping to control blood sugar levels and minimize complications for both the mother and the baby. Here are a few reasons why these procedures are important:

1. Carbohydrate Control:

   - Watch Your Carbohydrate Intake: The biggest influence on blood sugar levels comes from carbohydrates. It is essential to monitor and control carbohydrate intake throughout the day.

   - Choose Complex Carbohydrates: Opt for whole grains, fruits, vegetables, and legumes, which provide fiber and essential nutrients while causing a slower rise in blood sugar levels.

   - Limit Simple Carbohydrates: Minimize consumption of sugary foods and beverages, refined grains, and processed snacks that can cause rapid spikes in blood sugar.

2. Balanced Meals:

   - Eat Regularly: Space meals evenly throughout the day to help maintain stable blood sugar levels.

   - Include Protein: Incorporate lean protein sources such as poultry, fish, tofu, and legumes into meals and snacks to help stabilize blood sugar levels.

   - Healthy Fats: Include sources of healthy fats like avocados, nuts, seeds, and olive oil to promote satiety and support overall health.

3. Portion Control:

   - Watch Portion Sizes: Pay attention to portion sizes to avoid overeating and ensure balanced meals.

- Use Food Labels: Read food labels to understand serving sizes and carbohydrate content in packaged foods.

4. Meal Planning:

- Consistent Carbohydrate Intake: Aim for consistent carbohydrate intake at each meal to help regulate blood sugar levels.

- Meal Timing: Spread carbohydrate intake evenly throughout the day to prevent large fluctuations in blood sugar levels.

- Snack Smart: Include healthy snacks between meals to prevent dips in blood sugar and maintain energy levels.

5. Hydration:

- Drink Plenty of Water: Stay hydrated by drinking water throughout the day to support overall health and aid in blood sugar regulation.

6. Working with a Registered Dietitian:

- Individualized Plan: Consult with a registered dietitian specializing in gestational diabetes to create a personalized meal plan based on your specific needs and preferences.

- Monitoring Progress: Regularly review your dietary habits and blood sugar levels with your healthcare team to make necessary adjustments.

7. Physical Activity:

- Combine Diet with Exercise: Physical activity is an essential component of managing gestational diabetes. Incorporate regular exercise into your routine to improve blood sugar control and overall health.

By following these dietary recommendations and working closely with your healthcare team, you can effectively manage gestational diabetes and promote a healthy pregnancy outcome. It is crucial to prioritize nutrition, monitor blood sugar levels, and make lifestyle changes to support optimal health for both you and your baby.

Monitoring blood sugar level

Monitoring blood sugar levels and working closely with healthcare providers are essential components of managing gestational diabetes effectively. The following justifies the importance of these practices:

1. Blood Sugar Control: Regular monitoring of blood sugar levels allows you to track how your body responds to different foods, activities, and medications. By keeping your blood sugar levels within the target range recommended by your healthcare team, you can reduce the risk of complications for both you and your baby.

2. Individualized Care: Every pregnancy is unique, and each woman may respond differently to dietary changes, exercise, and medication. Working with healthcare providers, including obstetricians, endocrinologists, and registered dietitians, ensures that you receive personalized care tailored to your specific needs and circumstances.

3. Early Detection of Issues: Monitoring blood sugar levels regularly can help detect any fluctuations or abnormalities early on. This allows healthcare providers to make timely adjustments to your treatment plan, such as modifying your diet, exercise routine, or medication dosage, to maintain optimal blood sugar control.

4. Preventing Complications: Gestational diabetes increases the risk of complications during pregnancy and delivery, such as macrosomia (large birth weight), preterm birth, and preeclampsia. By closely monitoring

blood sugar levels and working with healthcare providers, you can minimize these risks and promote a healthier outcome for both you and your baby.

5. Education and Support: Healthcare providers can provide valuable education and support to help you manage gestational diabetes effectively. They can offer guidance on meal planning, exercise recommendations, blood sugar monitoring techniques, and emotional support to navigate the challenges of pregnancy with diabetes.

6. Collaborative Care: Managing gestational diabetes requires a multidisciplinary approach involving various healthcare professionals. By collaborating with your healthcare team, you can benefit from the expertise and insights of different specialists to optimize your care and ensure the best possible outcomes for you and your baby.

In conclusion, monitoring blood sugar levels and working closely with healthcare providers are essential strategies for managing gestational diabetes and promoting a healthy pregnancy. By staying proactive, informed, and engaged in your care, you can effectively control blood sugar levels, reduce the risk of complications, and support a positive pregnancy experience.

CHAPTER 7: VEGETARIAN AND VEGAN DIETS DURING PREGNANCY.

Meeting nutrient needs on a vegan diet.

Meeting nutrition needs on a vegetarian or vegan diet requires careful planning to ensure that you are getting all the essential nutrients your body needs. Here are some tips to help you meet your nutritional requirements on a plant-based diet:

1. **Include a Variety of Foods**: Eating a diverse range of fruits, vegetables, whole grains, legumes, nuts, seeds, and plant-based protein sources will help you obtain a wide array of nutrients.

2. **Focus on Protein**: Incorporate plant-based sources of protein such as beans, lentils, tofu, tempeh, edamame, quinoa, nuts, and seeds into your meals to meet your protein needs.

3. **Get Enough Iron**: Include iron-rich foods like lentils, chickpeas, spinach, tofu, pumpkin seeds, and fortified cereals in your diet. Enhancing iron absorption can be achieved by combining these foods with a vitamin C source.

4. **Ensure Sufficient Vitamin B12**: Since vitamin B12 is primarily found in animal products, consider taking a B12 supplement or consuming fortified foods like plant-based milks, cereals, or nutritional yeast.

5. **Include Omega-3 Fatty Acids**: Incorporate plant-based sources of omega-3 fatty acids such as chia seeds, flaxseeds, walnuts, and algae-based supplements to support heart and brain health.

6. **Calcium-Rich Foods**: Consume calcium-rich foods like fortified plant-based milks, tofu, almonds, leafy greens (such as kale and collard greens), and tahini to support bone health.

7. **Vitamin D**: Consider getting adequate sunlight exposure or taking a vitamin D supplement to support bone health, especially if you have limited sun exposure.

8. **Stay Hydrated**: Drink plenty of water throughout the day and consider incorporating hydrating foods like fruits and vegetables into your meals.

9. **Read Labels**: Check food labels for hidden animal-derived ingredients (e.g., gelatin, whey) and opt for plant-based alternatives when possible.

10. **Consult a Registered Dietitian**: If you have specific dietary concerns or health conditions, consider consulting a registered dietitian who specializes in vegetarian or vegan nutrition to create a personalized meal plan that meets your individual needs.

By following these tips and being mindful of your nutrient intake, you can maintain a well-balanced vegetarian or vegan diet that supports your overall health and well-being.

Plant-based sources of nutrients for pregnancy

During pregnancy, it is crucial to ensure that you are getting all the essential nutrients to support the healthy development of your baby and maintain your own well-being. While following a plant-based diet during pregnancy requires extra attention to nutrient intake, it is entirely possible to meet your needs through a variety of plant-based sources. Here are some key nutrients and their plant-based sources that are important during pregnancy:

1. **Folate**: Folate is essential for fetal development and helps prevent neural tube defects. Plant-based sources of folate include leafy greens (such as spinach, kale, and collard greens), lentils, chickpeas, asparagus, broccoli, avocado, and fortified cereals.

2. **Iron**: Iron is necessary for oxygen transport and blood production, especially during pregnancy when blood volume increases. Plant-based sources of iron include lentils, chickpeas, tofu, tempeh, soybeans, quinoa, pumpkin seeds, fortified cereals, and dark leafy greens like spinach and Swiss chard. Iron absorption can be improved by eating meals high in vitamin C along with foods high in iron.

3. **Calcium**: Calcium is crucial for bone development in the fetus and maintaining bone health in the mother. Plant-based sources of calcium include fortified plant-based milks (such as almond or soy milk), tofu made with calcium sulfate, almonds, tahini, figs, kale, collard greens, and fortified orange juice.

4. **Omega-3 Fatty Acids**: Omega-3 fatty acids are important for brain and eye development in the fetus. Plant-based sources of omega-3s include flaxseeds, chia seeds, walnuts, hemp seeds, algae-based supplements (like algae oil or seaweed), and enriched eggs or dairy alternatives.

5. **Protein**: Adequate protein intake is essential for fetal growth and development. Plant-based sources of protein include beans, lentils, chickpeas, tofu, tempeh, edamame, quinoa, nuts, seeds, and whole grains like brown rice and oats.

6. **Iodine**: Iodine is crucial for thyroid function and brain development in the fetus. Plant-based sources of iodine include iodized salt, seaweed (such as nori or kelp), and fortified plant-based milks.

7. **Vitamin D**: Vitamin D is important for calcium absorption and bone health. While sunlight exposure is a natural source of vitamin D, plant-based sources include fortified plant-based milks, fortified orange juice, and supplements.

8. **Vitamin B12**: Vitamin B12 is essential for nerve function and red blood cell production. Plant-based sources of vitamin B12 include fortified nutritional yeast, fortified plant-based milks, fortified cereals, and B12 supplements.

It's important to consult with a healthcare provider or a registered dietitian specializing in prenatal nutrition to ensure you are meeting your nutrient needs during pregnancy on a plant-based diet. They can provide personalized guidance and help you create a well-balanced meal plan that supports both your health and the health of your baby.

Potential supplements to consider for vegan mothers.

For vegetarian or vegan mothers, there are certain nutrients that may be more challenging to obtain from a plant-based diet alone. In these cases, supplements can be beneficial to ensure adequate intake of essential nutrients during pregnancy. Here are some potential supplements to consider for vegetarian or vegan mothers:

1. **Vitamin B12**: Vitamin B12 is primarily found in animal products, so it is important for vegetarian and vegan mothers to supplement with vitamin B12 to prevent deficiency. Red blood cell formation and nerve function depend on vitamin. Supplements can be in the form of cyanocobalamin or methylcobalamin, and they are available in tablet, capsule, or liquid form.

2. **Omega-3 Fatty Acids**: Omega-3 fatty acids, specifically DHA and EPA, are important for brain and eye development in the fetus. While plant-based sources like flaxseeds and walnuts provide ALA (a precursor to DHA and EPA), the conversion rate in the body is limited. In order to guarantee sufficient consumption of DHA and EPA, women who are vegetarians or vegans might want to think about taking omega-3 supplements based on algae.

3. **Iron**: Iron needs increase during pregnancy to support the increased blood volume and fetal development. Plant-based sources of iron may not be as readily absorbed as heme iron from animal products. Taking iron supplements can help avoid iron deficiency anemia. Ferrous sulfate or ferrous gluconate are common forms of iron supplements, but it's important to consult with a healthcare provider to determine the appropriate dosage.

4. **Calcium**: Calcium is crucial for bone development in the fetus and maintaining bone health in the mother. While plant-based sources of calcium are available, supplementation may be necessary if dietary intake is insufficient. Calcium carbonate or calcium citrate supplements can be considered under the guidance of a healthcare provider.

5. **Iodine**: Iodine is essential for thyroid function and brain development in the fetus. Plant-based sources of iodine may vary depending on the diet, so supplementing with iodine can help ensure adequate intake during pregnancy. Potassium iodide or kelp supplements are common forms of iodine supplements.

6. **Vitamin D**: Vitamin D is important for calcium absorption and bone health. While sunlight exposure is a natural source of vitamin D, supplementation may be necessary, especially for those living in areas with limited sunlight or during winter months. Vitamin D3 supplements derived from lichen or lanolin are suitable for vegetarians and vegans.

It's important for vegetarian and vegan mothers to consult with a healthcare provider or a registered dietitian specializing in prenatal nutrition before starting any supplements. They can assess individual nutrient needs, recommend appropriate dosages, and monitor nutrient levels throughout pregnancy to ensure optimal health for both the mother and the baby.

CHAPTER 8: WEIGHT MANAGEMENT DURING PREGNANCY.

Healthy weight gain for pregnancy

Healthy weight gain during pregnancy is essential to support the growth and development of the baby while also ensuring the mother's overall health and well-being. The pre-pregnancy weight and body mass index (BMI) of a woman determine how much weight she should gain during her pregnancy. Here are some broad recommendations for gaining weight during pregnancy that are healthful.

1. **Underweight (BMI less than 18.5)**:
   - Recommended weight gain: 28-40 pounds (about 13-18 kg)
   - Aim for a steady and gradual weight gain throughout pregnancy to support the baby's growth and development.

2. BMI 18.5-24.9 for normal weight:
"- Weight increase of 25–35 pounds (11–16 kg) is advised.

   - Focus on consuming a balanced diet rich in nutrients to support the nutritional needs of both the mother and the baby.

3. **Overweight (BMI 25-29.9)**:
   - Recommended weight gain: 15-25 pounds (about 7-11 kg)
   - Emphasize healthy eating habits and regular physical activity to manage weight gain and promote a healthy pregnancy.

4. **Individuals who are obese (BMI 30 or more) should aim to gain 11–20 pounds (5–9 kg).**
   - Work closely with healthcare providers to monitor weight gain and ensure proper nutrition and lifestyle choices.

Here are some additional tips for healthy weight gain during pregnancy:

- **Eat a Balanced Diet**: Focus on consuming a variety of nutrient-dense foods, including fruits, vegetables, whole grains, lean proteins, and dairy products. Avoid empty-calorie foods high in sugar and fat.

- **Remain Active:** As advised by your healthcare practitioner, partake in regular physical activity.

 Activities such as walking, swimming, prenatal yoga, and low-impact exercises can help maintain fitness levels and support healthy weight gain.

- **Monitor Weight Gain**: Keep track of your weight gain throughout pregnancy and discuss any concerns with your healthcare provider. Regular prenatal visits can help monitor your progress and address any issues that may arise.

- **Keep Yourself Hydrated:** To maintain general health and stay hydrated, sip lots of water throughout the day.

. Limit sugary beverages and opt for water, herbal teas, or other hydrating options.

- Pay Attention to Your Body: Eat when you're hungry and pay heed to your body's hunger cues. Restricting your food intake or missing meals can have a detrimental effect on your general health and energy levels.

- **Seek Support**: Talk to your healthcare provider, a registered dietitian, or a prenatal care specialist if you have questions or concerns about healthy weight gain during pregnancy. They can provide personalized guidance and support based on your individual needs.

By following these guidelines and making healthy choices throughout pregnancy, women can achieve appropriate weight gain that supports the health of both themselves and their growing baby. It's important to prioritize overall well-being and seek professional guidance when needed to ensure a healthy and successful pregnancy journey.

Managing weight gain and promoting healthy pregnancy

1. Eat a balanced diet: Maintain a balanced diet by emphasizing the consumption of a range of nutrient-dense foods, such as whole grains, fruits, vegetables, lean meats, and healthy fats. Steer clear of processed foods, sugary snacks, and foods high in fat in excess.

2. Monitor your weight: Keep track of your weight gain throughout your pregnancy and discuss any concerns with your healthcare provider. They can provide guidance on how to manage weight gain and make adjustments to your diet or exercise routine if necessary.

3. Stay active: Regular physical activity is important for managing weight gain during pregnancy. Aim for at least 30 minutes of moderate-intensity exercise most days of the week, such as walking, swimming, or prenatal yoga. Before beginning any new fitness regimen, make sure to speak with your healthcare physician.

4. Stay hydrated: Drinking plenty of water is essential for overall health and can help prevent excessive weight gain. Aim to drink at least 8-10 glasses of water per day and limit sugary drinks and caffeine.

5. Get enough sleep: Adequate rest is important for managing weight gain and promoting a healthy pregnancy. Aim for 7-9 hours of quality sleep each night and establish a relaxing bedtime routine to help you unwind before bed.

6. Manage stress: High levels of stress can contribute to weight gain and impact your overall health during pregnancy. Practice stress-reducing techniques such as deep breathing, meditation, or gentle exercise to help manage stress levels.

7. Seek support: Pregnancy can be a challenging time, so it's important to reach out for support when needed. Talk to your partner, friends, family, or a healthcare provider about any concerns or struggles you may be experiencing.

8. Attend regular prenatal appointments: Regular check-ups with your healthcare provider are essential for monitoring your weight gain, assessing your overall health, and addressing any concerns that may arise during pregnancy.

By following these strategies and working closely with your healthcare provider, you can effectively manage weight gain and promote a healthy pregnancy for both you and your baby.

Importance of physical activity and balanced diet

Physical activity plays a crucial role in conjunction with a balanced diet in managing weight gain during pregnancy. Regular exercise helps to burn calories, increase metabolism, and maintain muscle tone, all of which can contribute to a healthy weight gain during pregnancy. In addition, physical activity can help improve overall fitness, reduce the risk of gestational diabetes, lower blood pressure, and alleviate common pregnancy discomforts such as back pain and swelling.

When combined with a balanced diet, physical activity can enhance the benefits of healthy eating by promoting weight management, improving energy levels, and supporting overall well-being. Exercise also helps to regulate blood sugar levels, reduce stress, and boost mood, which are important factors for a healthy pregnancy.

It is important to consult with your healthcare provider before starting any exercise routine during pregnancy to ensure that it is safe and appropriate for your individual needs. By incorporating regular physical activity into your daily routine and maintaining a balanced diet, you can optimize your health and well-being during pregnancy while managing weight gain effectively.

CHAPTER 9: POSTPARTUM NUTRITION AND BREASTFEEDING

Nutritional needs during the postpartum period.

The postpartum period, also known as the postnatal period, refers to the time immediately following childbirth when a woman's body undergoes significant changes as it transitions back to its pre-pregnancy state. Proper nutrition during this time is crucial to support the healing process, replenish nutrient stores, promote recovery, and provide adequate nourishment for both the mother and her newborn.

Here are some key nutrition needs during the postpartum period:

1. **Caloric Intake**: While caloric needs vary depending on factors such as breastfeeding, physical activity level, and individual metabolism, most women require additional calories during the postpartum period to support healing and recovery. It is important to consume nutrient-dense foods to meet these increased energy needs.

2. **Protein**: Protein is essential for tissue repair and recovery after childbirth. Including lean sources of protein such as poultry, fish, eggs, legumes, nuts, and dairy products in your diet can help support healing and promote muscle recovery.

3. **Iron**: Iron levels may be depleted during pregnancy and childbirth, leading to an increased risk of iron deficiency anemia. Consuming iron-rich foods such as lean red meat, poultry, fish, beans, lentils, fortified cereals, and dark leafy greens can help replenish iron stores and prevent anemia.

4. **Calcium**: Calcium is important for bone health, especially during breastfeeding when calcium requirements are higher. Dairy products, fortified plant-based milks, tofu, almonds, and leafy greens are good sources of calcium that can help meet your daily needs.

5. **Fiber**: Adequate fiber intake is important for maintaining regular bowel movements and preventing constipation, which is common during the postpartum

period. Whole grains, fruits, vegetables, legumes, and nuts are rich sources of fiber that can support digestive health.

6. **Fluids**: Staying hydrated is essential for postpartum recovery and breastfeeding. Drinking plenty of water throughout the day can help prevent dehydration and support milk production.

7. **Omega-3 Fatty Acids**: Omega-3 fatty acids are important for brain development in newborns and may also help reduce inflammation and support overall health. Fatty fish such as salmon, chia seeds, flaxseeds, walnuts, and algae-based supplements are good sources of omega-3 fatty acids.

8. **Vitamins and Minerals**: Consuming a variety of fruits, vegetables, whole grains, nuts, seeds, and lean proteins can help ensure that you are getting a wide range of vitamins and minerals necessary for postpartum recovery and overall health.

It is important to consult with a healthcare provider or a registered dietitian to address any specific nutritional concerns or dietary restrictions during the postpartum period. By focusing on a balanced diet that includes a variety of nutrient-dense foods, you can support your body's healing process, replenish nutrient stores, and promote overall well-being during this important time.

Tips for supporting breastfeeding through proper nutrition

Supporting breastfeeding through proper nutrition during pregnancy is essential to ensure that both the mother and baby receive the necessary nutrients for optimal health and development. Here are some detailed tips for supporting breastfeeding through proper nutrition during pregnancy:

1. **Caloric Intake**: During pregnancy and while breastfeeding, a woman's caloric needs increase to support the growth of the baby and the production of breast milk. It is important to consume nutrient-dense foods to meet these increased energy requirements.

2. **Protein**: Protein is crucial for the production of breast milk and the growth and development of the baby. Including lean sources of protein such as poultry, fish, eggs, legumes, nuts, seeds, and dairy products in your diet can help support breastfeeding.

3. **Healthy Fats**: Healthy fats, such as omega-3 fatty acids, are important for brain development in the baby and can also help support milk production. Include sources of healthy fats like fatty fish (salmon, mackerel), avocados, nuts, seeds, and olive oil in your diet.

4. **Calcium**: Calcium is essential for bone health in both the mother and baby. Dairy products, fortified plant-based milks, tofu, almonds, and leafy greens are good sources of calcium that can support breastfeeding.

5. **Iron**: Iron levels may be depleted during pregnancy and childbirth, so it is important to consume iron-rich foods to prevent iron deficiency anemia. Lean red meat, poultry, fish, beans, lentils, fortified cereals, and dark leafy greens are good sources of iron.

6. **Fiber**: Adequate fiber intake is important for maintaining regular bowel movements and preventing constipation during pregnancy and breastfeeding. Fiber-rich foods include whole grains, fruits, vegetables, legumes, and nuts.

7. **Fluids**: Staying hydrated is crucial for milk production. Drinking plenty of water throughout the day can help prevent dehydration and support breastfeeding.

8. **Vitamins and Minerals**: Consuming a variety of fruits, vegetables, whole grains, nuts, seeds, and lean proteins can help ensure that you are getting a wide range of vitamins and minerals necessary for breastfeeding and overall health.

9. **Limit Caffeine and Alcohol**: Limiting caffeine intake and avoiding alcohol while breastfeeding is important to ensure the health and safety of the baby.

10. **Consult with a Healthcare Provider**: It is important to consult with a healthcare provider or a registered dietitian to address any specific nutritional concerns or dietary restrictions during pregnancy and breastfeeding.

By focusing on a balanced diet that includes a variety of nutrient-dense foods, you can support breastfeeding through proper nutrition during pregnancy and provide the best start for your baby's health and development.

Transition back to a regular diet after pregnancy

After pregnancy, returning to a regular diet is a crucial stage that needs to be carefully planned to guarantee that the mother and the unborn child continue to get the nutrients they need for optimum health. The following comprehensive advice can help you return to a regular diet after pregnancy:

1. **Gradual Transition:** It's critical to return to a regular diet gradually. By doing this, you assist your body adapt to the changes and lessen the chance of any discomfort or digestive problems.

2. **Balanced Diet**: Try to have a varied, well-balanced diet that is high in nutrient-dense foods. Fruits, vegetables, nutritious grains, lean meats, healthy fats, dairy products, and dairy substitutes should all be included in this.

3. **Caloric Needs**: Even while you might not require as many calories as you did during pregnancy and lactation, you should still consume enough calories to maintain your general health and energy levels. When your body tells you it's hungry, heed its signals and eat.

4. **Hydration**: It's critical for general health and wellbeing to stay hydrated. Throughout the day, sip on lots of water to keep your body hydrated and support its processes.

5. **Nutrient-Rich Foods**: Eat a diet high in nutrients to make sure you are getting all the vitamins and minerals you need. This can improve your postpartum recuperation and provide you more energy to take care of your infant.

6. **Protein**: Protein is important for tissue repair and muscle recovery post-pregnancy. Include lean sources of protein such as poultry, fish, eggs, legumes, nuts, seeds, and dairy products in your diet.

7. **Healthy Fats**: Healthy fats are essential for hormone production and overall health. Include sources of healthy fats like avocados, nuts, seeds, olive oil, and fatty fish in your diet.

8. **Iron-Rich Foods**: Consuming iron-rich foods is important, especially if you experienced blood loss during childbirth. Include sources of iron such as lean red meat, poultry, fish, beans, lentils, fortified cereals, and dark leafy greens in your diet.

9. **Calcium**: Calcium is important for bone health, especially if you are breastfeeding. Include sources of calcium such as dairy products, fortified plant-based milks, tofu, almonds, and leafy greens in your diet.

10. **Consult with a Healthcare Provider**: It is important to consult with a healthcare provider or a registered dietitian to address any specific nutritional concerns or dietary restrictions as you transition back to a regular diet after pregnancy.

You may help your recovery after giving birth and keep giving yourself and your child the best nutrition possible by concentrating on a balanced diet that consists of a range of nutrient-dense foods and making little adjustments over time.

Conclusion

"Prenatal Diets" is a comprehensive and informative guide that delves deep into the crucial role of nutrition during pregnancy. The book not only emphasizes the importance of maintaining a well-balanced diet for both the mother and the developing fetus but also provides a wealth of practical advice, meal plans, and recipes to help expectant mothers navigate their nutritional needs throughout the various stages of pregnancy.

One of the key strengths of "Prenatal Diets" is its focus on how different nutrients play a vital role in supporting the healthy growth and development of the baby. By explaining the significance of essential vitamins, minerals, and macronutrients, the book equips readers with the knowledge needed to make informed dietary choices that can positively impact their pregnancy journey.

Moreover, "Prenatal Diets" addresses common misconceptions and myths surrounding pregnancy nutrition, offering evidence-based information to help readers separate fact from fiction. By dispelling these myths and providing clear guidance on what foods to include and avoid during pregnancy, the book empowers expectant mothers to make educated decisions about their diet with confidence.

Additionally, "Prenatal Diets" encourages readers to seek personalized advice from healthcare professionals to tailor their dietary choices to their unique needs and preferences. By emphasizing the importance of individualized nutrition plans, the book underscores the importance of collaborating with healthcare providers to ensure optimal maternal and fetal health during pregnancy.

Overall, "Prenatal Diets" serves as an invaluable resource for expectant mothers looking to prioritize their nutrition and well-being throughout pregnancy. By following the expert guidance and practical tips provided in this book, readers can feel empowered to make positive choices that support their health and the healthy development of their baby, setting the foundation for a successful and fulfilling pregnancy journey.